FIRST STEPS IN AROMATHERAPY

Jane Dye

First Steps in Aromatherapy

A Simple and Straightforward
Guide, Listing 58 Essential Oils

Index compiled by
Lyn Greenwood

SAFFRON WALDEN
THE C.W. DANIEL COMPANY LIMITED

First published in Great Britain in 1996
by The C.W. Daniel Company Limited
1 Church Path, Saffron Walden,
Essex CB10 1JP, England

ISBN 0 85207 292 9

Designed by Peter Dolton.
Designed and produced in association with
Book Production Consultants plc,
25–27 High Street, Chesterton
Cambridge, CB4 1ND England.
Typeset by Cambridge Photosetting Services,
Cambridge, England.
Printed in England by
St. Edmundsbury Press, Bury St. Edmunds, Suffolk.

Contents

Jane Dye is the author of *Aromatherapy for Women and Children*, a widely successful book now available worldwide – written to help clarify the conflicting advice available about the many and varied uses of essential oils and their safety. Jane runs a busy health food shop and aromatherapy practice and has shared her experiences in aromatherapy through her writing, broadcasting and through her work. She likes to stress the important role that self help has to play in the treatment of any condition, whilst clarifying when to seek professional advice, be it orthodox or complementary.

Jane initially trained as a Sports Therapist and went on to be trained by Robert Tisserand, who is recognised worldwide as a leading authority on aromatherapy. Together they founded the Tisserand Aromatherapy Institute to provide comprehensive training, education, publishing and research.

Jane and husband Tom, a writer/musician, live with their daughter Josie and various animals on the edge of Northumberland National Park and the Cheviot Hills.

For Tom, Josie and Michael.

Heartfelt thanks go to Michael Green, Anna Gregory and everyone at Hanny's, especially Shirley, Sharon, Martin, Tim and Andrea. My love and thanks go to my family of friends – from Tony and Lali, Rafa and Jake, to those upstairs – for making me smile again, inside and out and without whom getting this far would have been impossible.

With all my heart I especially thank Tom and Josie – whose love, understanding and encouragement make all things possible.

Take time to smell the roses...

Introduction

Aromatherapy continues to be the fastest growing complementary therapy. More and more case studies are being recorded, proving the effectiveness of essential oils for therapeutic use. The increasing respect that aromatherapy commands from the general public, hospitals and medical centres all over the world speaks for itself, as more and more people benefit from this gentle, subtle yet highly effective therapy. Aromatherapy can be a simple practice, it is natural, uncomplicated and it works – beautifully.

Aromatherapy is also big business, involving scientists and professionals from all disciplines. Aromatic sources are cultivated on an ever-increasing scale to cope with demand and, as demand increases, so does the necessity for high standards of quality control, clarity of marketing and professional training. To practice aromatherapy professionally one needs in-depth comprehensive study and application – but for those with no training there are still many oils which can be used with total confidence and assurance of a positive benefit. The most valuable thing about aromatherapy is that it is for everyone – young or old, male or female – as long as there is a physical, mental or emotional need for benefit, there is always an essential oil that can help.

I am lucky enough to have a busy health food shop and aromatherapy practice in one of the most spectacular places in Britain, in terms of both the scenery and the people. The cross section of customers and clients I meet is one of the widest and most interesting I could wish for. I meet those who come in for themselves, for their friends, partners, children or families; for their livestock and their pets – but every person has one thing in common – they have all either heard of, seen or experienced the profound benefits that can be gained from the use of essentials oils – and they want to learn to use it for themselves.

We all surely prefer a natural, effective treatment that causes no added stress to our systems. Every day we become more aware of the complications that synthetically produced medicines can cause, especially during pregnancy and for children and babies. Synthetic drugs can also suppress the symptoms, rather than treating the cause, thus adding stress to the system which can lead to adverse side effects, allergic reaction or dependency. For those who wish to be directly involved with their own self help – for those who prefer a remedy that treats the whole system rather than just the symptoms – aromatherapy provides a safe and natural treatment, one that I know from my own experience can often produce surprising results where other methods of treatment have failed.

Aromatherapy can be used alongside orthodox or other alternative medicines, and if used with understanding and respect can help to establish and maintain health and well being in a safe, non-toxic and non-habit forming way. It is a particularly successful therapy for any stress related conditions from eczema to depression, whilst the physiological benefits of some of the oils are second to none. Tea tree essential oil is a classic example and is known as the "Medicine Kit in a Bottle". It is used in a wide range of products to combat all manner of ailments from pulmonary infection to cold sores, and is invaluable in its highly antiseptic, antifungal use. (It should be the law of the land that every home keep Tea Tree oil and Lavender oil in the medicine kit.)

There are three basic areas of aromatherapy.

Clinical Aromatherapy is practised in France by the medical profession, where its role is commonly accepted. G.P.s prescribe essential oils, usually for internal use, for a wide range of infections and disease, using oils of the highest quality.

Aesthetic Aromatherapy is generally used as an adjunct to beauty therapy and relaxation. Ready blended oils help to create a general feeling of wellbeing. This is most commonly available through Beauty Clinics.

Holistic Aromatherapy brings the complete healing process together and is practised by professionally trained aromatherapists. This involves in-depth assessment of the individual, to recognise and evaluate subtle weaknesses and physical and emotional symptoms. Treatment is given after lifestyle, diet and nutrition, exercise and general physical and emotional wellbeing have all been thoroughly considered. For home use, other than general assessment and obvious conditions, specific diagnosis should only be made by a professional. Treatment has a profound and far reaching influence so keep to the guidelines given in the book to start with.

It has to be said that this is a simple, straightforward guide to the first steps in aromatherapy; there are many conditions that you can treat and help with just a basic knowledge. Once you get into the subtleties of making your own blends a whole new world of possibilities opens up. One quarter of a drop of a particular essential oil can shift the whole emphasis of a blend – but that is another story, so read on. If you do wish to take it further then there are many short, intermediate and fully professional courses available, one of which is bound to suit the level of proficiency you desire; useful addresses are given at the end of the book.

In the meantime, let me remind you – the most valuable thing about aromatherapy is that it is for everyone – young or old, male or female – as long as there is a physical, mental or emotional need there is always an essential oil that can help.

CHAPTER ONE

So what is this "Aromatherapy"?

The actual term "aromatherapy" was coined by René Gattefossé, a French chemist who published the first book on the subject in 1928. This fired great response and much research into the medicinal benefits of the essential oils, particularly in France and Italy. Dr Jean Valnet, a French doctor and army surgeon, contributed most to the scientific validity of aromatherapy, using the oils to great effect to treat burns and wounds during the second world war. However, the Austrian biochemist Marguerite Maury was the great force in establishing the reputation of the therapy. She dedicated the majority of her life to researching the oils and demonstrating their effects on the nervous system, their rejuvenating properties, the theory of individual prescription and the holistic approach to the therapy. M Gattefossé and Mme Maury's books both make fascinating reading. Robert Tisserand wrote the first general introduction to the subject in English in 1977, having set up the first UK essential oil business in 1974, selling essential oils to the general public. Since then demand has grown beyond all expectation and oils are readily available. As with suppliers, there are possibly even more choices in training courses now available in this country. Robert and I set up the Tisserand Aromatherapy Institute in 1987, to establish comprehensive and qualified aromatherapy training and a focus for professional research and interest. The last few years have seen a phenomenal increase in the information available on aromatherapy, not just to specialists, but to everyone, and Robert Tisserand and the Institute continue to play a leading role.

The origins of aromatherapy go back centuries. The use of plants and herbs is the oldest method of healing disease and pain, and the magical and medicinal properties of plants have been recorded in the oldest writings in history, in myth and folklore. Essential oils are used in thousands of litres in present times by the food, pharmaceutical and perfume industries. Virtually everything used today in modern drugs can be traced back to botanical extract. Hippocrates said that there is a remedy for everything to be found in Nature; most of us would like to believe this too, if only we could find a positive way to reconnect with the wonders Nature has to offer us. Aromatherapy can help us to do this and to help ourselves. We are capable of anything with a little help!

The World Health Organisation made a pronouncement as long ago as 1974, saying that if the Third World was to achieve adequate health care by the year 2000, then they would have to retrieve their herbal traditions and nurture and develop their traditional systems of medicine, rather than rely on expensive western drugs and chemicals. This now applies more than ever before and not just to the Third World. Don't forget though, whatever your beliefs, both orthodox and complementary treatments are valid and make sense and as long as the treatments are safe and effective – well, the choice is yours.

Aromatherapy is a natural healing therapy using essential oils to improve physical, mental and emotional wellbeing. Only when our vital organs, our nervous and circulatory systems are relaxed and unstressed can we be at ease in mind, body and spirit and begin to boost our own natural resources to heal ourselves in a natural way.

Essential oils are extracted from single botanical sources, from the part of the plant yielding the maximum amount of essential oil. Some are easy to extract such as Rosemary, others costly. Jasmine, like Rose and Neroli (orange blossom oil), is highly prized due to the huge amount of petals needed to extract a tiny amount of oil, (thousands of petals to make one drop), and the high labour costs involved in the delicate harvesting of the petals. To extract the oil, known as an absolute, a special method is used.

An absolute is very concentrated; the odour and therapeutic properties are very strong, therefore only very small amounts are ever needed to give the same benefit as larger amounts of oils distilled in the standard way. Absolutes are also sold extracted in a carrier oil, usually Jojoba. So bear this in mind when you are told the price. If you can afford these oils, you will have a very precious investment. As with any essential oils never buy a synthetic copy, and especially with these very special oils, always buy from the best supplier you can.

Bear in mind the same crop may be cultivated under differing conditions in different parts of the world and the oils available vary considerably in quality and cost. There are many cheap and chemical copies of essential oils available too, some even mixed with pure oil, but these are not recommended for therapeutic use. As a general rule, you get what you pay for. A reputable supplier with a high turnover is more likely to supply fresh stock with quality control from source to shelf. Essential oils do have a shelf life – some for years, others for only a few months, so don't be tempted to buy cheap oils unless you just want perfume. The best suppliers will also always have help and advice readily available and a wide range of good products to get you started.

Although called essential oils, pure oils should not feel oily unless they have been diluted. Aromatherapy can be incredibly subtle yet highly powerful and the most appealing aspects of its use are the many and varied methods of application.

So, how do you use these amazing essential oils?

CHAPTER TWO

Safety first

Some oils are toxic in certain circumstances. A reputable supplier will only sell these oils to a professional therapist and will wish to see and verify his or her qualifications before so doing. This is one of the ways in which a good supplier can maintain some degree of safety in the use of essential oils available to the general public. Some essential oils are toxic in excess but the ones we cover in this book are the most commonly used and are not on the toxic list. They are undiluted though, so remember they are very concentrated. "Less is more" in aromatherapy.

Here are some important points to remember:

1. *Never use oils undiluted, apart from Lavender or Tea Tree in special circumstances.*

2. *Never take the oils internally.*

3. *Never use oils near the eyes.* (If ever any essential oil is splashed into the eyes, wash with plenty of cool water. If any stinging persists, seek medical advice.)

4. *Never massage directly over skin infection, inflammation, varicose veins, recent fractures or scar tissue, or when fever or temperature is present.*

5. *Don't use the oils on babies under 1 month old. Only use Lavender, Roman Chamomile or Tea Tree up to 7 years.*

Dosage for Babies and Children:

1 month to 6 months	*1 drop in 10 mls of carrier oil*
6 months to 18 months	*2 drops in 10 mls*
18 months to 7 years	*3 drops in 10 mls*
7 years to 14 years	*4 drops in 10 mls*
(See methods of use)	

6. *If pregnant, avoid the use of the following oils:*

> *Clary Sage*
> *Geranium*
> *Jasmine*
> *Juniper*
> *Peppermint*
> *Rose*
> *Rosemary*

(If you do feel any of the above oils may be of help whilst pregnant, consult a fully qualified professional aromatherapist, as some can be of great benefit in certain circumstances.)

7. *If in any doubt, consult a fully qualified professional aromatherapist.*

CHAPTER THREE

Methods of use

Essential oils elicit an effect or reaction – be it physical, mental, emotional or spiritual. When applied to the skin, research has shown that the essential oils are absorbed into the system via the bloodstream and circulated to all parts of the body. During this process they also release their own natural properties such as plant hormones. Some oils also have an affinity with certain organs in the body, such as Juniper which has a particular affinity with the kidneys.

In addition, smelling the oils has a strong influence on our mind and emotions. An olfactory message is sent directly to the brain each time you smell anything – be it pleasant or otherwise, consciously or not. This direct reaction affects mood, memory and emotion and causes response in our central nervous system and brain. Touch and smell are our "close range" senses and aromatherapy powerfully combines the therapeutic benefits of both, causing a deep response.

Application includes massage, inhalation, baths, compresses, creams, diffusers/vaporisers or any method of smelling the oils, from a couple of drops in the hoover bag to a drop on the pillow. The most beneficial and long lasting benefit is when the oils are first diluted in a carrier oil and applied by massage, as this is when the two most fundamental senses of touch and smell are combined to maximum effect.

Touch and smell are not only biologically the earliest to develop but also the most evocative of all our senses. From the moment of birth an infant uses these senses to identify and bond with the mother thus ensuring nourishment, protection and survival. So from the very beginning, these senses have a basic role to play in communication. As we move into adulthood, body contact decreases as communication by action and word takes over, yet the stresses of everyday living increase. If these stresses and strains are allowed to continue, an imbalance occurs, immunity decreases and ill health results. Aromatherapy helps to restore balance; as it works on many levels, the therapy is highly versatile in treating all manner of conditions. Babies, children and animals respond very well to the therapy, (although not necessarily in that order!) – their responses being free from any pre-conceived ideas or expectations. They respond favourably to a loving touch – as do all of us. It is the most natural thing in the world.

Massage:

For basic massage, movements should generally be towards the heart, lighter over bone and firmer over muscle and in a clockwise direction over the stomach. At all times use a smooth, even pressure. There are many books and courses available, but trust your own sensitivity and intuition when giving a massage – no two people are alike in their responses to touch or odour – all have different needs and wishes. Read their reactions, gain their trust and help them to "breathe out", relax and enjoy.

The language of touch is as difficult to describe as the language of smell, but the pleasure from early skin contact continues throughout our lives – as we get older our ability to value touch increases yet the opportunity can decrease as touch becomes loaded with social implications. This ability to value touch, sensitivity, pleasure and trust should not be lost in adulthood when some are not touched at all, socially or otherwise and can lose a very great source of wellbeing. Skin satisfaction is one of the most important of experiences, skin being, after all, the largest organ in the body, with 50 nerve endings, hundreds of sensory perceptors, 3 million cells and over 100 sweat glands for *every* square inch of skin – quite something!

Of the many types of body contact therapies massage is the most common, and an aromatherapy massage makes the most effective use of essential oils. Massage can stimulate and relax muscles, improve circulation and encourage lymph flow, improve digestion, and thus boost physical and mental balance and wellbeing and help towards maintaining a healthy immune system. The benefits of massage are countless – with essential oils, almost limitless.

For use in massage, essential oils are blended with a vegetable, nut or seed oil which should preferably be cold pressed, this avoiding any chemical processes. ("Baby oil" is usually mineral and is not absorbed into the skin.)

Essential oils should be pure and undiluted. They are very concentrated, so always use them diluted in a carrier oil. The only two essential oils you can use on the skin neat are Lavender and Tea Tree.

Carrier oils:

Almond	most used and suitable for all skin types.
Avocado	heavy, green, rich in Vit A & E.
Grapeseed	palest green and for use on all skins.
Jojoba	waxy oil, solidifies in cold temperatures.
Peach Kernal	light oil, ideal for facial massage or more delicate skins.
Wheatgerm oil	high in Vit. E. *CAUTION*: may cause reaction in those who have a wheat allergy. Patch test first, leaving for 24 hours.

There are many other oils you can use, but always use cold pressed if you can and always vegetable.

Dosage:

The usual blend of essential oil to carrier oil is 2–3%, which works out at ½ drop to 1 ml of carrier oil

1 drop to 2 mls etc ...

In other words, divide the number of mls of carrier/base oils by 2, to give you the number of drops of essential oils to use.

Avoid blending more than you need at the time as the oils lose their therapeutic value once oxidised and do not keep for as long.
e.g. (small teaspoonful carrier oil = 4 mls):

4 mls = 2 drops of essential oil
10 mls = 5 drops
20 mls = 10 drops etc.

Don't use the oils on babies under 1 month old. Only use Lavender, Roman Chamomile or Tea Tree up to 7 years.

Dosage for Babies and Children:

1 month to 6 months	*1 drop in 10 mls of carrier oil*
6 months to 18 months	*2 drops in 10 mls*
18 months to 7 years	*3 drops in 10 mls*
7 years to 14 years	*4 drops in 10 mls*

Bath:

Run the bath to the required temperature, close the door and windows. Add the essential oils, making sure you "swish" the surface of the water to disperse them before you get in. Lie back, soak away and breathe deeply – this is your time to spoil yourself.

For babies and children refer to the appropriate dosage for their age and apply the amount of drops given to a full-sized bath. Take care to ensure essential oils are not splashed into eyes.

Dosage for Adults:

10–12 drops of pure essential oil to a full size bath.
Use up to a combination of 4 different oils.
Add vegetable oil as well if you wish, to help nourish the skin.
Avoid rubbing it all off again with a towel – pat gently and go and put your feet up if you can.

Inhalations:

Inhalations are second to none for any pulmonary/respiratory conditions as the oils* are absorbed directly where they are needed most and give maximum benefit.

1. *Steam Inhalation:*
To about half a pint of just-boiled water add the oil(s), cover your head and container with a towel, close your eyes and breathe deeply.

Dosage:

2 to 3 drops of essential oil
Repeat several times or as required.
(Some only like 1 drop although a friend's 80-year old Granny can manage 5 drops of Tea Tree and she doesn't come up for air inside 5 minutes!)
*See Tea Tree

2. *Direct Inhalation:*

One or two drops of essential oils can be put on a handkerchief or tissue and sniffed when desired. This is instantly effective and can help with anything from nerves to exhaustion. It is very handy for tiredness when driving, studying, or any situation when the brain needs a kick-start and equally soothing for when you want to calm down – before an interview, visiting the dentist, exams, a driving test or coping with life's general pace …

*Gargle:**

2 to 3 drops in half a glass of water. Swish thoroughly between each gargle as essential oils do not mix readily in water.

Compress:

Use a piece of clean absorbent material – a clean handkerchief, sterilised flannel or cotton wool. Add the essential oils to cooled, previously boiled water, peppermint or chamomile tea, (chilled or warm, depending on the treatment). "Swish" the oils over the surface to mix well. Soak the oils off the surface of the liquid using the material. Apply to affected area for at least 10 minutes. For stomach or back pain where a warm compress is required, a hot water bottle on top of the compress will give added relief. For a cold compress, use a medical freezer pack, crushed ice, (inside a plastic bag to keep everything dry), or a bag of frozen

*See Tea Tree

vegetables. (Peas are best as they mould to the area well.)

Dosage:
Up to 10 drops per half pint of liquid.

Don't use the oils on babies under 1 month old. Only use Lavender, Roman Chamomile or Tea Tree up to 7 years old.

Air Freshener:
All essential oils are anti-bacterial, some more than others. For use as an air freshener, place a few drops in the hoover bag before hoovering, a colourless essential oil on the radiator, on the carpet or on linen, or on a light bulb ring. These fit over the light bulb and have a small lip onto which you place a few drops of your favourite oil. As the light bulb heats up the ring the vapours are released from the essential oil. This is an inexpensive and very effective method of combating airborne bacteria and freshening a room, and the oils are useful mood enhancers as well.

Dosage:
Some oils have a very strong odour so only use one drop at first. You probably won't notice much of a smell after a while, as you get used to it. If you aren't sure, go outside, clear your nose and come back in again. You want to avoid knocking your visitors out with the strength of smell.

Diffusers/Vaporisers:

There are many types available, all specifically made for using essential oils. The oils are usually gently heated by candle or electricity and the vapours released into the atmosphere. They should always be made of an inflammable material as essential oils are flammable, so again always buy from a reputable supplier. They are usually heated by electricity or candle flame, although I personally think the "Aromastream" is the most effective, as although electric, air is fanned through a porous "filter" onto which you can place various oils. It is safe and very effective and you really get your money's worth from your precious oils. Because of its design it is safe to leave on if you are not in the room.

For a home-made vaporiser, you can add steaming water to oils and let the steam waft the oils around the room that way. This is particularly effective in a sick-room as the oils you use can be anti-bacterial and healing as well as soothing and comforting. **CAUTION**: If using this method in a child's room, be sure you guard the hot water well.

Scalp/Hair Treatments:

Essential oils can be very effective in treating scalp conditions, from dandruff to lice and lots in between. Some treatments, especially for head lice in children, can be unpleasant or uncomfortable to use so try an aromatherapy treatment instead. For children, let them help in preparing the blend so they feel involved.

Method:

Make up the appropriate blend using 2–3%
dilution as normal, in a base/carrier oil of your
choice. Remember to adjust the strength of
blend for children. Massage well into the scalp.
Leave for a minimum of 30 minutes and up to
2 hours. For maximum effect, a cap over the
head and a towel or soft hat on top of that will
increase the temperature and aid the treatment. Massage neat shampoo into the hair
after the required length of time and then
wash in the normal way.

For dandruff add the essential oils to the
shampoo using the same dilution.

Ointments and Creams:

To make an ointment or cream, add appropriate essential oils to a non-fragranced base
for antiseptic, nourishing, perfume creams or
ointments – or be adventurous and make
your own.

For 30 mls:

> *7 g unrefined beeswax*
> *23 mls vegetable oil**
> *15–20 drops of essential oil*

Method:

Place the shredded beeswax and vegetable oil
in a heat proof bowl inside a pan of water over
a gentle heat. Stir until the wax has melted.
Place the bowl into a pan of cold water, adding

*For a more nourishing blend, in place of 23 mls of
vegetable oil, you could use 20 mls of Almond Oil or Peach
Kernel with 3 mls of Avocado/Jojoba/Wheatgerm oil.

the essential oils as it begins to thicken, mixing well.

This makes a more solid cream which softens when applied to the warmth of the skin. Lavender, Tea Tree and Bergamot in equal proportions makes a good antiseptic cream.

For a thinner cream ideal for face or body, don't use the beeswax and use half the quantity of vegetable oil, but add rose or orange flower water instead.

Always use clean equipment and glass containers. Don't forget to label and date your lotions and potions.

Foot Bath:

Use as for Compress, adding the essential oils to cooled, previously boiled water, peppermint or chamomile tea, (chilled or warm, depending on the treatment). "Swish" the oils over the surface to mix well and soak your feet for as long as you feel comfortable – Bliss!

Buying and Storage of Essential Oils and Products:

When you have found a good supplier, you will find there are many products available that make life for the "newly initiated" very much easier, in addition to a wide range of pure and organic essential oils and carrier/base oils. Some additional products available are as follows:

Light Bulb Rings
Massage Rollers

Mini Kits – usually containing small samples of essential oils

Pre-Blended products for a variety of moods and benefits

Massage Oils

Lotions/Creams

Bath Oils

Soaks

Shower Gels

Shampoos

Conditioners

Hair Treatments

Antiseptic/Healing Creams

Antiseptic/Healing Lotions

Antiseptic/Healing "Wipes"

Soothing and Cooling Gels

Books

Advice – this being vital and a good sign of the standards offered by your supplier

Boxes in which to keep your collection of essential oils

Essential oils do have a shelf life, some for years and some for only months, so always ensure you buy your pure essential oils from the best supplier. They should be stored away from heat and light, and in darkened, glass, airtight bottles. As well as being very volatile, essential oils can oxidate and turn cloudy, so always put the tops back on firmly and as quickly as you can. Look after them, and they will do the same and more for you.

CHAPTER FOUR

Blends

Essential oils are known to have "base", "middle" or "top" notes which play an important part in any blend. Those with a strong base note are longer lasting but not immediately perceived and are good fixatives. The more uplifting and refreshing oils are generally those with a strong top note and a sharper more perceived odour which tends to fade more quickly.

A good blend is like a piece of music – with a good bass (base) note to hold the blend together, a sound middle and a zing in the treble (top) note for initial impact and response. The most effective blends should always include a good balance of essential oils with top, middle or base notes for optimum benefit and long lasting fragrance. If using oils for a physical problem, for example, also include an oil or oils for emotive response and if using 3 oils, don't choose all three with top notes or it will be too "skinny" and won't last well – or all with base notes because it will be too "heavy" and overpowering. Avoid using more than three oils in a blend to start with.

Essential oils generally fall within the categories shown below, although always remember that the oils affect the whole system and many uses and benefits overlap although there are subtle differences. Getting to know these subtleties is half the delight. Cross reference by reading the complete physical, mental and emotional profiles given for each particular essential oil.

CHAPTER FIVE

List of Oils by Property

Antidepressant
Clary Sage
Jasmine
Neroli
Ylang Ylang

Antiseptic
Bergamot
Eucalyptus
Geranium
Juniper
Sandalwood
Tea Tree

Balancing/Regulating
Geranium

Decongestant
Eucalyptus
Peppermint
Tea Tree

Detoxifying
Juniper
Rosemary

Diuretic
Benzoin
Chamomile
Clary Sage
Frankincense
Geranium
Juniper
Rosemary
Sandalwood

Antifungal
Tea Tree

Aphrodisiac
Clary Sage
Jasmine
Neroli
Rose
Sandalwood
Ylang Ylang

Calmative
Chamomile
Frankincense
Lavender
Neroli
Rose
Ylang Ylang

Disinfectant
Bergamot
Juniper
Lavender
Tea Tree

Euphoric
Clary Sage
Jasmine

Expectorant
Benzoin
Eucalyptus
Sandalwood

Fortifying
Frankincense
Rosemary

Rejuvenating
Frankincense

Soothing
Chamomile
Frankincense
Sandalwood
Ylang Ylang

Strengthening
Rosemary
Sandalwood

Toning
Rose
Rosemary
Sandalwood

Refreshing
Bergamot
Peppermint
Rosemary

Sedative
Chamomile
Clary Sage
Lavender
Neroli
Sandalwood

Stimulating
Black Pepper
Peppermint
Rosemary

Warming
Benzoin
Black Pepper
Peppermint

CHAPTER SIX

Essential Oils
A–Z

BENZOIN – *styrax benzoin*
Reminder: Soothing, penetrating

Origin:
Thailand/Java/Sumatra
From the gum of the tree.

Colour:
Reddish brown

Odour – base

Warming, drying, comforting and rich in odour with a hint of sweetness – a good fixative in a blend.

Benzoin is particularly helpful in tense, "cold" conditions, both physically and emotionally. Because of its warming properties Benzoin can be a very positive oil and can help in creating a "padded zone" between us and events.

Physical:
Arthritis – bronchitis – colds – coughs – infections – influenza – gout.

Emotional:
Despair – loneliness – negativity – sadness – stress.

Applications:
Air Freshener / Bath / Compress / Diffuser / Vaporiser / Massage.

BERGAMOT – *citrus bergamia*
Reminder: A smile inside

Origin: **Colour:**
Sicily   Yellow/Green
From the fruit of the tree.

Odour – top

Rich/citrus/sweet and refreshing. Bergamot is an oil
known to uplift the spirits and inspire. Like most
other citrus oils it is a notable antiseptic, yet is more
refreshing than sharp being slightly sweet. It is a
very versatile oil and appeals to both sexes.
Bergamot is a classic ingredient of Eau de Cologne.

Physical:
Bergamot is particularly effective in treating skin
conditions: acne – boils – blisters – cold sores –
eczema – herpes – psoriasis – known to have a regulating effect on digestive system (under/over eat-
ing) – shingles – urinary problems.

Emotional:
Can allay anger – anxiety – depression – despair /
despondency. Good for lack of confidence – lack of
courage – nervous tension – worry.

***CAUTION:**
Although Bergamot is of special use in skin conditions it also increases photosensitivity of the skin for
up to 3 hours, so avoid direct sunlight or sunlamps
after use, as pigmentation of the skin may result.
Bear in mind that this also applies to many commercially produced toiletries and perfumes which
include bergamot oil. (It is also added to Earl
Grey Tea!)

Applications:
Air Freshener / Bath / Compress / Diffuser /
Vaporiser / Massage.

BLACK PEPPER –
piper nigrum
Reminder: Hot & penetrating

Origin:
India – and one of the
earliest spices known to
man. (It was a highly
prized luxury and was
used to pay taxes.) From
the berries of the plant.

Colour:
Usually amber

Odour – middle

Black Pepper is hot, penetrating, spicy and strong,
so only a little is ever needed and can be very effective in helping any conditions of mind or body
where warmth is needed. It can help to stimulate
the circulation and is useful for restoring tone.

Physical:
Good for anaemia – arthritis – cellulite – chilblains –
constipation – cramp – muscular aches and pains –
stiffness – water retention.

Emotional:
Fatigue – indifference – lethargy – melancholy.

Applications:
Air Freshener / Bath / Compress / Diffuser /
Vaporiser / Massage.

***CAUTION:
Black Pepper is strong so use sparingly.

CEDARWOOD – *cedrus atlantica*
Reminder: Composure/Strength

Origin: ***Colour:***
Morocco   Clear
From the wood of the tree.

Odour – base

Warm, rich, woody and fortifying and a good fixative in a blend. Cedarwood is "warm and dry" and can help many skin conditions. The odour is attractive to both sexes and is a popular ingredient in perfumes and toiletries.

Physical:
Bronchitis – catarrh – coughs – dandruff* – general tonic – oily skin.

Emotional:
Helps to compose and focus thoughts – Gives strength in stressful conditions.

Applications:
Air Freshener / Bath / Compress / Diffuser / Vaporiser / Massage.

* see scalp/hair treatment.

CHAMOMILE:
ROMAN – *anthemis nobilis*
GERMAN – *matricaria chamomilla*
Reminder: Anti-inflammatory

Colour:

Blue or Yellow. (It can stain, so take care.)

Origins:

Roman – England, from the flowers of the plant. This is nearly always cultivated, the herb commonly grown as a lawn. (Buckingham Palace has a fine example – apparently.)

German – France, from the flowers and seeds. German chamomile is known as the true chamomile and tends to grow wild. This has a higher level of azulene in its make up, giving a darker blue colour and a stronger aroma and is subsequently of more benefit in aromatherapy.

Odour – middle

Mellow, sweet, hay-like. (Chamomile is of more use physically than emotionally and so blends with more emotive oils.)

Physical:

Aches & pains – acne – arthritis – colic – cramps – dermatitis – dull aches & pains – eczema – feverish conditions – inflammation – menstrual & menopausal pain – nervous upsets – psoriasis – rashes – rheumatic and gout pains – scabbing – skin eruptions – sprains – swelling – teething.

Emotional:

Chamomile can often help to break the vicious circle of tension and effect by its physical benefits.

Applications:

Air Freshener / Bath / Compress / Diffuser / Vaporiser / Massage.

CLARY SAGE – *salvia sclarea*
Reminder: release

Origin:
France
From the flowering tops
of the herb.

Colour:
Pale Yellow/Clear

Odour – middle

Nutty, floral and slightly sweet and can have a profoundly soothing action in cases of nervous tension for both men and women. Clary Sage is also particularly helpful for women due to its affinity with the uterus and is consistent in helping those who suffer from PMT/PMS. It is very helpful along with Jasmine and Geranium during labour and post-natally.

Physical:
Use it to help during birth – for high blood pressure – menopause – mental/sexual debility – premenstrual and menstrual problems – stress.

Emotional:
Anxiety – depression – mental/sexual debility – post natal depression – menopause – moodiness – negativity – panic – pre-menstrual and menstrual tensions – restlessness – worry – stress.

Applications:
Air Freshener / Bath / Compress / Diffuser / Vaporiser / Massage.

CAUTION:
Clary Sage can make some feel exceptionally relaxed and "at ease" – avoid alcohol, driving or having to concentrate directly after a treatment.

CYPRESS –
cupressus sempervirens
Reminder: Astringent

Origin:
France
From the leaves and cones
of the tree.

Colour:
Clear/Pale Yellow

Odour – middle/top

Refreshing, woody and spicy, with a hint of pine.
Cypress blends well with more emotive oils.

Physical:
Cypress is one of the most astringent essential oils.
It is effective on cellulite – dandruff* (with oily scalp)
– foot perspiration – oily skin – general perspiration
– haemorrhoids – PMS/PMT – varicose veins. (Never
massage directly over veins. Gently stroke the blend
above the vein and towards the heart.)

Emotional:
Cypress is more physical than emotional in its uses.

Applications:
Air Freshener / Bath / Compress / Diffuser /
Vaporiser / Massage.

* see scalp/hair treatment.

EUCALYPTUS –
eucalyptus globulus
Reminder: Respiratory

Origin: *Colour:*

Spain   Clear

From the leaves of the tree.

Odour – top

Fresh, powerful and long lasting, so use sparingly.

Physical:

Asthma – bronchitis – catarrh – colds – coughs –
headaches due to congestion – influenza – sinusitis
– sore throats. Eucalyptus is an effective decongestant and expectorant. (Eucalyptus is also a good
insect repellent.)

Emotional:

Eucalyptus is more physical than emotional in
its use.

Applications:

Air Freshener / Bath / Compress / Diffuser /
Vaporiser / Inhalation / Massage.

FRANKINCENSE –
boswellia thurifera
Reminder: Deep & profound/a breath out

Origin:
Somalia
From the gum of the tree.

Colour:
Clear/Pale Yellow

Odour – middle/base

Fresh, green and woody with a little sweetness and a hint of pine. Long lasting in any blend.

Physical:
Frankincense has more use emotionally and spiritually than physically, however it is invaluable in a blend for its fortifying properties. It is also good for ageing skin.

Emotional:
Lack of inner strength/faith/confidence/courage – good for anger – apprehension – bad dreams/ disturbed sleep – when feeling "little" inside – lost or alone – fear – grief – hopelessness – insecurity – irritability – nervous tension – remorse/dwelling on past events – stress – tearfulness – vulnerability – weakness – worrying thoughts.

Frankincense gives a "spiritual cuddle" and should not be underestimated in its value. It has been used for centuries as an aid to meditation and a comfort to those who dwell in the past or who suffer anxiety or hurt from past events. Use it when a "breath out" is needed.

Applications:
Air Freshener / Bath / Compress / Diffuser / Vaporiser / Massage.

GERANIUM – *pelargonium odoratissimum/graveolens*
Reminder: Balance

Origin: *Colour:*
Egypt   Palest green
From the flowers and
leaves.

Odour – top

Fresh, very green, slightly rosy scent. Geranium mixes well with most oils. This is a very useful oil to regulate physical, mental and emotional imbalances/extremes and despite its subtle neutrality should not be underestimated.

Physical:

Addiction – cellulite – chilblains – circulation – congestion (as in cleansing the system of accumulated toxins) – constipation – fluid retention – gastritis – hormone imbalances (especially post natal) – menopausal problems – PMS/PMT – Skin dry/oily.

Emotional:

Anxiety – confusion – depression – lethargy – mood swings – hyper/hypoactivity – tearfulness.

Applications:

Air Freshener / Bath / Compress / Diffuser / Vaporiser / Massage.

***CAUTION:

Due to its hormonal action, Geranium should not be used by the lay person during pregnancy. Consult a professional aromatherapist if you feel this oil may be of help to you during pregnancy.

JASMINE –
jasminum officinale & grandiflorum
Reminder: Deep, warm, euphoric

Origin: **Colour:**
India   Dark yellow/orange
From the petals of the bush.

Odour – strong top, middle and base notes

Deep, exotic, heady and sensual and adds an extra special dimension to any blend.

Jasmine, like Rose and Neroli oil, is highly prized. Jasmine Absolute is very concentrated, the odour and therapeutic properties being very strong. Only very small amounts are ever needed to give equal benefit to other distilled essential oils, hence it is also sold diluted in a carrier oil, usually Jojoba, which is fine for home use. It mixes beautifully with any blend, especially anything citrus, as these oils lose their impact in a short time, yet Jasmine just goes on and on …

Physical:

Jasmine is invaluable during childbirth as it has a strong action on and affinity with the uterus, aiding contractions yet easing pain. It is second to none as an aid to labour and is particularly effective with Clary Sage and Geranium (and/or Rose/Neroli depending on the circumstances). Jasmine can also give a real "lift" when spirits are low or when one is tired or weary.

Emotional:

Jasmine is an effective anti-depressant – aphrodisiac – euphoric. Good for apathy – depression – despair/despondency – frigidity/impotence – lethargy – lack of enthusiasm – post natally – sexual debility – shyness.

Jasmine can have a great influence on everyone. Its mellow and warming actions on emotional levels go hand in hand with its physical benefits of relaxing and rounding out tenseness and rigidity – it is commonly compared with the effect of an exceedingly good bottle of champagne!

Applications:

Air Freshener / Bath / Compress / Diffuser / Vaporiser / Massage.

***CAUTION**:

Do not use Jasmine whilst pregnant, until labour begins, then it becomes invaluable. In addition to its profoundly therapeutic properties, Jasmine can help to create the most beautiful atmosphere for giving birth.

JUNIPER – *juniperis communis*
Reminder: Eliminates toxins

Origin:
Italy
From the berries of the
bush.

Colour:
Clear

Odour – middle

Balsamic and woody with a hint of pine. Juniper is very effective in that it can promote excretion of uric acids, waste products and excess toxins in our systems and helps in purifying the blood.

Physical:
The clearing/detoxifying aspect of Juniper helps with arthritis – cellulite – chilblains – congestion – constipation – cramp – cystitis. Good as a diuretic – helps with gout – hangover – headaches – PMS/PMT – urinary infection – water retention.

Emotional:
Clears and purifies the atmosphere and nerves. Good for those who care for others.

Applications:
Air Freshener / Bath / Compress / Diffuser / Vaporiser / Massage.

***CAUTION:**
Because of its action on the kidneys, Juniper should not be used during pregnancy.

LAVENDER –
lavandula officinalis
Reminder: Healing

Origin: *Colour:*

France   Clear or pale yellow

From the flowering tops.

Odour – middle

Sweet, floral and slightly woody. Although it has a strong smell initially, usually a sign that the odour doesn't last long, Lavender lasts well in any blend being particularly healing on the mind, body and emotions. Every home in the land should keep a bottle of Lavender within easy reach – it being the most commonly used essential oil.

Physical:

Lavender is second to none for burns. If applied immediately, Lavender can prevent any blistering or scarring and will speed up natural healing of any wound as it stimulates cell renewal. It can also be a great aid to sleep, another great healer!

Abscess – acne – aches & pains – arthritis – bites – blisters – boils – bruises – burns – chickenpox – chilblains – colic – cuts – cystitis – dermatitis – eczema – headache (tension) – heat rash – immune system stimulant – insect bites – insomnia – measles – nappy rash – nausea – neuralgia – PMT/PMS – rashes – scalds – scarring – sciatica – shingles – skin disorders – sores – sprains – spots – stiffness – stings – stretch marks – sunburn – teething – wounds.

Emotional:

Anger – anxiety – fear – fright – hysteria – hyper-activity – impatience – insomnia – irritability – jealousy – negative thoughts – nervousness – panic – paranoia – post-natally – restlessness – shock – stress – tension – worry.

Applications:

Air Freshener / Bath / Compress / Diffuser / Vaporiser / Massage / Neat.

*****CAUTION:**

Whilst Lavender can be used undiluted on specific areas such as spots and burns, it can sometimes sting a little, so patch test first.

NEROLI/ORANGE
BLOSSOM – *citrus aurantium*
Reminder: Anti-Stress

Origin: *Colour:*
Tunisia   Yellow
From the flowers of the
bitter orange tree.

Odour – middle/top

Richly floral, refreshing and reviving – slightly haunting and peaceful.

Neroli is a very special oil, as in addition to its physical use it has profound influence in treating any stress-related conditions. Because most "dis-ease" comes from stress, be it physical, mental, emotional or spiritual, Neroli is valuable in most blends.

Neroli, like Jasmine and Rose oil, is highly prized and although costly only a little is ever needed for great effect. It is invaluable for treating stress or shock in either male or female.

Physical:

Broken veins – fatigue – headaches – hypertension – nervous tension (as in diarrhoea / indigestion / insomnia) – palpitations – panic – scarring – skin sensitivity / dryness / ageing – skin blemishes – stretch marks.

Emotional:

A good aphrodisiac and euphoric. Soothes anger – anxiety. Helps with despondency – distress – emotional depression – nervous exhaustion – frustration – grief – hopelessness – irritability – nervous tension – PMS/PMT & associated emotions – shock – stress – tearfulness – vulnerability.

Applications:

Air Freshener / Bath / Compress / Diffuser / Vaporiser / Massage.

PEPPERMINT – *mentha piperita*
Reminder: Cool cleansing

Origin: *Colour:*
Brazil   Pale Yellow
From the leaves.

Odour – top

Cool, fresh & very much of peppermint. Peppermint is a very strong oil with an overwhelming odour. Although used in a wide variety of commercially available products care should be used with dosage.

Physical:
Peppermint is invaluable against nausea and travel sickness. Also good for neuralgia, indigestion and hot and tired feet.

Emotional:
Stimulant.

Applications:
Air Freshener / Bath / Compress / Diffuser / Vaporiser.

CAUTION:
Although excellent for nausea, peppermint should not be used during pregnancy due to its stimulating properties.

ROSE – *rosa damascena/otto*
Reminder: Queen of emotions

Origins:
Bulgaria
From the petals.

Colour:
Reddish brown

England – Phytol*

(*Phytols are the inspiration of Peter Wilde who is responsible for a completely new method of essential oil extraction – one which is attracting much interest and attention. The process is carried out at room temperature or less and does not involve steam or heat or alcohol, resulting in an essential oil without any solvent residues and which is very true to nature. Rose Phytol is considered much purer and stronger than oils produced by conventional methods. We are famous all over the world for our roses – organic English rose oil is now a reality.)

Odour – middle/base

Intensely floral, heady and rich. Rose, Jasmine and Neroli are very special essential oils and although expensive only a little is needed for great effect.

Physical:

Addiction – allergies – birth – constipation – hangover – headache (toxins) – migraine (toxins) – menopausal problems – PMT/PMS. Rose can also help to promote menstruation and regulate flow as it has a particular affinity with the reproductive system. It is of great benefit to sensitive, mature or hard skin. It can have a gentle toning effect on capillaries and can help with thread veins.

Emotional:

Bereavement – bewilderment – despair/despondency – grief – hopelessness – loneliness – negativity – post-natal depression – regret – sadness – sorrow.

Applications:

Air Freshener / Bath / Compress / Diffuser / Vaporiser / Massage.

CAUTION:

Because of its particular affinity with the female reproductive system, Rose should not be used during pregnancy. If you feel this oil may help you, contact a fully qualified professional aromatherapist.

ROSEMARY – *rosemarinus officinalis*

Reminder: Stimulation

Origin:	***Colour:***
Spain	Clear
From the leaves.	

Odour – middle/top

Fresh, cleansing, penetrating and "herbaceous".

Physical:

Aches (muscular) – brain inactivity – bruises – chilblains – coldness (circulation) – colds – congestion – constipation – cramp – dandruff (dry, itchy scalp) – exhaustion (physical) – hangover – inertness – laziness – lethargy – memory loss – muscular tension – sluggishness – stiffness – tiredness.

Emotional:

Apathy – confusion – day dreaming – "hibernation" – indecision – listlessness – memory loss – mental fatigue – negativity – procrastination.

Applications:

Air Freshener / Bath / Compress / Diffuser / Vaporiser / Massage.

CAUTION:

Do not use Rosemary during the first 4 months of pregnancy. If you do feel that you would like to use Rosemary whilst pregnant, and after the first 4 months, then contact a fully qualified professional aromatherapist.

SANDALWOOD –
santalum album
Reminder: Fortifying

Origin: *Colour:*
India   Pale Yellow
From the wood of the tree.

Odour – base

Slightly sweet, woody, rounded and enduring.
Sandalwood is a very popular oil to use in a blend
because of its fortifying and enduring qualities. It is
a good fixative, has over 150 compounds and blends
well with most oils.

Physical:

Aphrodisiac, (physical tonic with affinity for reproductive organs) – back pain, (related to kidneys and
adrenals) – exhaustion – immunity stimulant
(action on the spleen in aiding white blood cell
production) – influenza – laryngitis – lumbago – skin
antiseptic (good for teenage males, along with Tea
Tree) – sore throat.

Emotional:

Aphrodisiac, (widespread reputation from its use as
a perfume) – apprehension – exhaustion – fear –
humility – emotional insecurity – lack of courage –
sensitivity – shyness – tearfulness – timidity – weakness of spirit.

Applications:

Air Freshener / Bath / Compress / Diffuser /
Vaporiser / Massage.

TEA TREE –
melaleuca alternifolia
Reminder: Antiseptic/antifungal

Origin: *Colour:*
Australia   Clear
From the leaves of the tree.

Odour – middle/top

Tea Tree has a strong medicinal, warm, spicy and fresh odour.

There has been a very great deal published on the many and varied exceptional therapeutic benefits of Tea Tree; this is not at all surprising as Melaleuca Alternifolia is undoubtedly one of the most remarkable of Nature's gifts. Whole books have been published on this oil alone, but I will try to keep it brief! Suffice it to say, everyone should have a bottle of Tea Tree. It is inexpensive and highly effective and quite rightly known as the "Medicine Kit in a Bottle". Even though highly antiseptic, antiviral and antifungal, (a study by Penfold in 1925 showed Tea Tree to be 12 times stronger than carbolic acid), it is still a natural, non-addictive, non-toxic and safe medicine to be appreciated by all.

Tea Tree can be used neat on specific areas such as spots, cold sores, warts & verrucas.

Physical:
Abscess – acne – asthma – arthritis – athlete's foot – boils – bronchial congestion – burns – candida albicans – catarrh – chickenpox – cold sores – colds – colic – congestion – coughs – cystitis –dandruff – dermatitis – disinfectant – eczema – expectorant – foot odour – hair care – haemorrhoids – head lice – heat rash – herpes – inflammation – influenza – insect bites & stings (insect repellent) – infected gums – infection – measles – oral hygiene – parasites – rashes – respiratory congestion – ringworm –

shingles – sinusitis – skin disorders (dermatitis, eczema, psoriasis, seborrhoea) – sore throat – spots – stings – sunburn – tonsillitis – toothache – verrucas – viral conditions – warts.

Tea Tree is second to none for anything pulmonary, respiratory – colds, influenza, sore throat etc., and is especially effective in clearing sinusitis. Use the inhalation method to get straight to the area needing treatment. Use it as often as required and at a comfortable strength.

Applications:
Air Freshener / Bath / Compress / Diffuser / Gargle / Mouth wash / Inhalation / Massage / Vaporiser.

N.B. It is interesting to note that New South Wales is where Tea Tree is grown, and also the only place, (thankfully!) where the potentially lethal Funnel Web spider lives – to which Tea Tree is an effective antidote. It has unique chemistry in that it contains trace constituents not found anywhere else in Nature.

YLANG–YLANG –
cananga odorata
Reminder: Exotic

Origin:
Philippines
From the blossom of the
tree. (Translated it means
"flower of flowers".)

Colour:
Pale Yellow

Odour – middle/base

Sweet, richly exotic, particularly heady and sensual. Ylang Ylang has a very strong odour and can be overpowering, so only a little is needed. It blends particularly well with the "skinnier" odours of most citrus oils. It is known as the poor man's Jasmine.

Physical:
High blood pressure – palpitations.

Emotional:
Soothes anger – aphrodisiac – boosts confidence – good for detachment – emotional insecurity – frustration – introversion – jealousy – sensitivity – sexual debility – stubbornness.

CAUTION:
Because of its particularly "heady" aroma, Ylang Ylang, (pronounced "eelang"), is not suitable for those who are prone to headaches.

CHAPTER SEVEN

List of Symptoms A–Z

ABSCESS –
Lavender/Tea Tree

ACHES & PAINS –
Chamomile/Juniper/Lavender/Rosemary

ACNE –
Bergamot/Chamomile/Lavender/Tea Tree

ADDICTION –
Geranium/Rose

ANGER –
Frankincense/Lavender/Neroli/Ylang Ylang

ANTIDEPRESSANTS –
Geranium/Jasmine/Neroli/Sandalwood

ANTISEPTIC –
Bergamot/Tea Tree

ANXIETY –
Bergamot/Clary Sage/Geranium/Lavender/
Neroli/Rose

APATHY –
Jasmine/Rosemary

APHRODISIACS –
Jasmine/Neroli/Sandalwood/Ylang Ylang

APPREHENSION –
Frankincense/Sandalwood

ARTHRITIS –
Benzoin/Black Pepper/Chamomile/Juniper/
Lavender/Tea Tree

ASTHMA –
Eucalyptus/Tea Tree

ATHLETES FOOT –
Tea Tree/Lavender

BACTERIA –
Tea Tree

BEREAVEMENT –
Frankincense/Neroli/Rose

BIRTH –
Clary Sage/Geranium/Jasmine/Neroli/Rose

BITES –
Lavender/Tea Tree

BLISTERS –
Bergamot/Lavender/Tea Tree

BLOOD PRESSURE (see hypertension)

BLUES –
Bergamot/Geranium/Jasmine/Neroli

BOILS –
Bergamot/Lavender/Tea Tree

BROKEN VEINS –
Neroli/Rose

BRONCHITIS –
Benzoin/Cedarwood/Eucalyptus/Tea Tree

BRUISES –
Black Pepper/Lavender/Rosemary

BURNS –
Lavender/Tea Tree

CANDIDA ALBICANS –
Tea Tree

CATARRH –
Cedarwood/Eucalyptus/Tea Tree

CELLULITE –
   Black Pepper/Cypress/Geranium/Juniper

CHICKENPOX –
   Bergamot/Lavender/Tea Tree

CHILBLAINS –
   Black Pepper/Geranium/Juniper/Lavender/
   Rosemary

CIRCULATION –
   Geranium/Rosemary

COLDS –
   Benzoin/Eucalyptus/Rosemary/Tea Tree

COLD SORES –
   Tea Tree

COLIC –
   Chamomile/Lavender/Tea Tree

CONFIDENCE –
   Bergamot/Frankincense/Sandalwood

CONFUSION –
   Cedarwood/Geranium/Rosemary

CONGESTION –
   Cedarwood/Geranium/Rosemary

CONSTIPATION –
   Black Pepper/Geranium/Juniper/Rosemary

COUGHS –
   Benzoin/Cedarwood/Eucalyptus/Tea Tree

COURAGE –
   Bergamot/Frankincense/Sandalwood

CRAMP –
   Black Pepper/Chamomile/Juniper/Rosemary

CUTS –
   Lavender/Tea Tree

CYSTITIS –
   Juniper/Lavender/Tea Tree

DANDRUFF –
Cedarwood/Cypress/Rosemary/Tea Tree

DEPRESSION –
Benzoin/Bergamot/Clary Sage/Jasmine/Neroli/
Sandalwood

DERMAL INFLAMMATION –
Chamomile/Tea Tree

DERMATITIS –
Chamomile/Lavender/Tea Tree

DESPAIR/DESPONDENCY –
Benzoin/Bergamot/Jasmine/Neroli/Rose

DETOXIFYING –
Juniper/Rosemary/Tea Tree

DIGESTION –
Bergamot/Neroli

DISINFECTANT –
Tea Tree

DIURETIC –
Juniper

DREAMS (and sleep) **–**
Frankincense/Lavender/Neroli

DYSPEPSIA (see indigestion)

ECZEMA –
Bergamot/Chamomile/Lavender/Tea Tree

EMOTIONS – (under/over-emotional)
Geranium/Lavender/Neroli/Rose/Ylang Ylang

ENERGY – (under/over-energetic)
Bergamot/Geranium/Jasmine/Lavender/
Rosemary

EUPHORICS –
Bergamot/Jasmine/Neroli

EXHAUSTION –
Neroli/Rosemary/Sandalwood

EXPECTORANTS –
Eucalyptus/Tea Tree

FATIGUE –
Black Pepper/Neroli/Rosemary

FEET –
Cypress/Peppermint/Tea Tree

FEMININITY –
Jasmine/Neroli/Rose/Ylang Ylang

FLEAS –
Tea Tree

'FLU – (see influenza)

FLUID RETENTION –
Geranium/Juniper/Rosemary

FOCUS –
Cedarwood/Clary Sage/Rosemary

FRIGIDITY –
Jasmine/Neroli/Rose/Ylang Ylang

FRUSTRATION –
Benzoin/Lavender/Neroli/Ylang Ylang

FUNGI – (see athletes foot/verrucas)

GARGLES –
Tea Tree

GERMAN MEASLES –
Bergamot/Chamomile/Lavender/Tea Tree

GOUT –
Benzoin/Black Pepper/Cypress/Juniper/
Lavender

GRIEF –
Frankincense/Neroli/Rose

GUILT –
Benzoin/Cedarwood/Frankincense/Rose

HAEMORRHOIDS –
Cypress/Tea Tree

HANGOVER –
Juniper/Rose/Rosemary

HEADACHES –
Eucalyptus/Juniper/Lavender/Neroli/Rose

HEAD LICE –
Tea Tree

HEAT BUMPS/RASH/PRICKLY HEAT –
Bergamot/Lavender/Tea Tree

HERPES –
Tea Tree (see cold sores)

HOPELESSNESS –
Frankincense/Neroli/Rose/Sandalwood

HORMONES –
Geranium/Rose

**HYPERTENSION/HIGH BLOOD
PRESSURE –**
Neroli/Ylang Ylang

IMMUNITY –
Lavender/Sandalwood

INDIGESTION –
Peppermint

INFECTIONS –
Benzoin/Bergamot/Tea Tree

INFLAMMATION –
Chamomile/Lavender/Tea Tree

INFLUENZA –
Benzoin/Eucalyptus/Lavender/Sandalwood/
Tea Tree

INSECT BITES/STINGS –
Bergamot/Lavender/Tea Tree

INSECT REPELLENT –
Citronella/Eucalyptus/Tea Tree

INSOMNIA –
Clary Sage/Lavender/Neroli/Rose

IRRITABILITY –
Lavender/Neroli/Ylang Ylang

JEALOUSY –
Lavender/Ylang Ylang

LARYNGITIS –
Sandalwood/Tea Tree

LETHARGY –
Black Pepper/Geranium/Jasmine/Rosemary

LONELINESS –
Benzoin/Rose/Sandalwood

LUMBAGO –
Black Pepper/Rosemary/Sandalwood

LUNGS –
Eucalyptus/Tea Tree

MEASLES –
Bergamot/Lavender/Tea Tree

MELANCHOLIA –
Benzoin/Bergamot/Rose/Sandalwood

MEMORY –
Rosemary

MENOPAUSE –
Chamomile/Clary Sage/Geranium/Rose

MENSTRUATION –
Chamomile/Clary Sage/Geranium/Juniper/
Rose

MENTAL FATIGUE –
Cedarwood/Rosemary

MOOD SWINGS –
Clary Sage/Geranium/Sandalwood

MUSCLES (aches & pains) –
Black Pepper/Chamomile/Lavender/Rosemary

NAPPY RASH –
Chamomile/Lavender/Tea Tree

NAUSEA –
Lavender/Peppermint

NEGATIVITY –
Benzoin/Clary Sage/Jasmine/Neroli/Rose

NERVOUS CONDITIONS –
Bergamot/Chamomile/Lavender/Neroli

NETTLE RASH –
Bergamot/Lavender/Tea Tree

NEURALGIA –
Lavender/Peppermint

NITS (see head lice)

OEDEMA –
Chamomile/Geranium/Juniper/Rosemary

PANIC –
Clary Sage/Lavender/Neroli

PERIODS (see menstruation)

PERSPIRATION –
Cypress

PILES (see haemorrhoids)

PMS/PMT
(Pre-menstrual syndrome/tension)
Clary Sage/Cypress/Geranium/Juniper/
Lavender/Neroli/Rose

POST-NATAL PERIOD –
Geranium/Jasmine/Lavender/Rose/
Sandalwood

PRICKLY HEAT –
Lavender/Tea Tree

PSORIASIS –
Bergamot/Chamomile/Lavender/Tea Tree

PULMONARY CONDITIONS –
Eucalyptus/Tea Tree

RASHES –
Chamomile/Lavender/Tea Tree

REGRET –
Frankincense/Rose/Sandalwood

REGULATING OIL –
Geranium

RELAXATION –
Clary Sage/Frankincense/Jasmine/Lavender

RESPIRATORY CONGESTION –
Eucalyptus/Tea Tree

RESTLESSNESS –
Bergamot/Clary Sage/Lavender/Neroli

RHEUMATISM (see arthritis)

RINGWORM –
Tea Tree

RUBELLA (see measles)

SADNESS –
Benzoin/Bergamot/Jasmine/Rose

SCABS –
Lavender/Tea Tree

SCALDS –
Lavender/Tea Tree

SCARRING –
Lavender/Neroli

SCIATICA –
Chamomile/Lavender

SENSITIVITY –
Geranium/Rose/Sandalwood/Ylang Ylang

SHINGLES –
Bergamot/Lavender/Tea Tree

SHOCK –
Lavender/Neroli

SHYNESS –
Jasmine/Sandalwood

SINUS –
Eucalyptus/Tea Tree

SKIN –
DRY – Geranium/Lavender/Neroli
OILY – Cedarwood/Cypress/Neroli
MATURE – Frankincense/Lavender/Neroli/
Rose
PROBLEM – Lavender/Sandalwood/Tea Tree

SLEEP –
Lavender

SORES –
Lavender/Tea Tree

SORROW –
Benzoin/Neroli/Rose

SPOTS –
Bergamot/Lavender/Sandalwood/Tea Tree

SPRAINS –
Chamomile/Lavender

STIFFNESS –
Black Pepper/Lavender/Rosemary

STINGS –
Bergamot/Lavender/Tea Tree

STRESS –
(Massage) – Cedarwood/Clary Sage/
Frankincense
Jasmine/Lavender/Neroli/Rose

STRETCH MARKS –
Lavender/Neroli

SUNBURN –
Lavender/Tea Tree

SWELLING (see oedema)

TEARFULNESS –
Geranium/Frankincense/Neroli/Rose/
Sandalwood

TEETHING –
Chamomile/Lavender

TENSION –
Clary Sage/Frankincense/Lavender/Neroli/
Rosemary

THROAT (sore throat) –
Eucalyptus/Sandalwood/Tea Tree

THRUSH – see candida albicans

TIREDNESS –
Jasmine/Rosemary

TONSILLITIS –
Tea Tree

VARICOSE VEINS –
CYPRESS/LAVENDER/ROSEMARY
(Never massage below the vein, always
between the vein and the heart)**

VERRUCAS –
Tea Tree

VIRUS –
Tea Tree

VOMITING (see nausea)

VULNERABILITY –
Benzoin/Cedarwood/Frankincense/Neroli/
Sandalwood

WARTS –
   Tea Tree

WATER RETENTION –
   Black Pepper/Geranium/Juniper/Rosemary

WEAKNESS –
   PHYSICAL – Sandalwood
   EMOTIONAL – Cedarwood/Frankincense/
   Sandalwood

WORRY –
   Benzoin/Bergamot/Clary Sage/Frankincense/
   Lavender

CHAPTER EIGHT

List of the more commonly used Essential Oils

The following is a list of the more commonly used essential oils of the 250 or so used in aromatherapy today. Because of the subtle nature of aromatherapy and the overlapping uses of essential oils it is not possible to describe their benefits fully in only a few words – but as an approximate guide, a very brief description is given alongside each one to give an indication of their general use.

The essential oils profiled in this book in more detail have been marked with an asterisk.

BASIL –
ocimum basilicum – herb.
Spicy aroma. Clears the mind – restorative, positive, tonic. Good for focus and alertness.

*BENZOIN –
styrax benzoin – resin.
Warm, soothing oil – both physically and emotionally. Good for those with fears and stresses, who feel they can't cope – encourages a feeling of contentment and warm relaxation.

*BERGAMOT –
citrus bergamia – rind of fruit.
Refreshing, joyous and uplifting, Bergamot gives a delicate lightness and brightness to

most blends and situations. A very encouraging oil for good cheer. Helpful for many skin conditions.

*BLACK PEPPER –
piper nigrum – fruit/spice.

Warm and stimulating, especially good for muscular aches and pains – a very solid, secure oil that can help to counteract many negative situations.

CAJEPUT/CAJUPUT –
melaleuca leucadendron – tree.

Stimulating and reviving oil – good for toothache, colds, respiratory infections (via inhalation) and head lice.

***CAUTION – can irritate.

CAMPHOR –
cinnamomum camphora – wood.

Acts as tonic – good for depressive states. Respiratory/circulatory stimulant. May be helpful with stiff muscles.

CARAWAY –
carum carvi – seed.

Overall tonic but use with caution.

***CAUTION – can irritate.

CARROT SEED –
daucus carota – seed.

Cleansing and toning – can help with liver, kidney problems due to its diuretic properties.

*CEDARWOOD –
cedrus atlantica – wood.

General tonic with a powerful calming and

soothing effect on the mind and emotions. Gives strength and focus and a feeling of self worth. Can be good for respiratory congestion.

CELERY –
apium graveolens – seeds.

Tonic oil, useful for digestion. Can also help with water retention and cellulite.

*CHAMOMILE –
matricaria chamomilla/anthemis nobilis – herb/flower.

Anti-inflammatory, soothing and calming essential oil – good for any "angry" situations – injury, sprains, teething and similar. A very peaceful oil, calm and quiet.

CINNAMON –
cinnamomum zeylanicum – tree.

A very strong antiseptic. It is tonic and warming in its effect – can promote circulation. ***CAUTION** – powerful and should be used with care.

CITRONELLA –
cymbopogon nardus – grass.

Best known as an insect repellent, but can also help to clear the mind.

*CLARY SAGE –
salvia sclarea – herb.

Best known for its effect in easing PMT/PMS and for its affinity with the reproductive system. Can also be a euphoric and a highly positive oil for both sexes.

CLOVE –
eugenia caryophyllata – tree.

Well known localised pain reliever, especially effective for toothache.

CORIANDER –
coriandrum sativum – seed.

A warming stimulant, said to have effect on digestion and spleen.

CUMIN –
cuminum cyminum – herb.

Stimulant – warming and good for toxic congestion.

*CYPRESS –
cupressus sempervirens – tree.

Powerful astringent and a known tonic.

DILL –
anethum graveolens – herb.

Good for digestive disorders/discomfort.

*EUCALYPTUS –
eucalyptus globulus – tree leaves.

Antiseptic, antiviral and can help with congestions and fever.

FENNEL –
foeniculum vulgare – herb.

Fennel has effective cleansing and toning properties and is known for its use as a diuretic. Can help increase milk flow.

*FRANKINCENSE –
boswellia thurifera – gum.

Known for its calming and comforting

effect on the nervous system and for its revitalising effect on skin. Good for stressful situations.

*GERANIUM –
pelargonium graveolens/ odoratissimum – plant.

Geranium is best known for its regulating, balancing and harmonising properties – it is also cleansing and refreshing with a mild tonic action.

GINGER –
zingiber officinale – root.

Warm, spicy, dry and known for its stimulating properties, ginger is good for muscular aches and pains and digestive disorders.

GRAPEFRUIT –
citrus paradisi – rind of fruit.

Grapefruit is known for its tonic action – a very cleansing and revitalising oil.

HYSSOP –
hyssopus officinalis – flowers.

Stimulates alertness and clarity and can have a regulating effect on the circulation, digestion and lungs.

*JASMINE – *jasminum officinale/graniflorum – flowers.*

Highly exotic and sensual, a very beautiful essential oil well known for its aphrodisiac and uplifting properties. A noted euphoric and relaxant.

*JUNIPER –
juniperus communis – berry.

A well known diuretic, good for toxic congestion (esp. liver and kidneys). Can help with cellulite and arthritic conditions.

*LAVENDER –
lavandula officinalia – herb.

The classic remedy for burns and any situation where new cell growth is required. Can also help with relaxation and insomnia. A very healing and harmonising oil.

LEMON –
citrus limonum – fruit.

A refreshing, cleansing and uplifting oil. An effective tonic.

LEMONGRASS –
symbopogon citratus – herb.

Known for its tonic properties and antiseptic uses.

LIME –
citrus aurantifolia – fruit.

Refreshing, uplifting and a general tonic.

LINDEN BLOSSOM –
tilia europaea – flowers.

A delicate and unique fragrance and a luxurious natural perfume. Linden Blossom is known for its relaxing properties.

MANDARIN –
citrus madurensis – fruit.

Mandarin is a calm and gentle oil, ideal for use on the very young or old or anyone feeling fragile. It is gently uplifting in its properties, with a use in skin preparations.

MARJORAM –
origanum majorana – herb.

A known calming and comforting essential oil. Good for tension, strain, (muscular or emotional) and stress.

MAY CHANG –
litsea cubeba – fruit.

Good for use where astringent and toning properties are needed – sweet and fruity fragrance.

MELISSA –
melissa officinalis – herb.

Melissa is a known nerve tonic and its gentle action is both calming and uplifting.

MYRRH –
commiphora myrrha – resin.

Soothing, drying and antiseptic, myrrh is good for certain skin conditions and mouth ulcers.

NIAOULI –
melaleuca viridiflora – tree.

Known to be effective for problem skin due to its antiseptic properties. Can help to fortify immune system with special reference to the respiratory system.

*NEROLI –
citrus aurantium – flowers.

Neroli is the classic anti-stress essential oil. Good for skin.

NUTMEG –
myristica fragrans – tree.

Nutmeg is a very stimulating and invigorating essential oil.

***CAUTION** – Nutmeg is not recommended for home use.

ORANGE –
citrus aurantium – fruit.

Refreshing and uplifting. Can be an effective skin tonic.

OREGANO –
origanum vulgare – herb.

Oregano can have a beneficial effect on the digestive and respiratory systems.

***CAUTION** – not recommended for home use.

PALMAROSA –
cymbopogon martini – grass.

Refreshing and clarifying, palmarosa is also used in soaps and many skin preparations.

PARSLEY –
petroselinum sativum – herb.

Parsley is a strong diuretic.

***CAUTION** – not for home use.

PATCHOULI –
pogostemon patchouli – herb.

Relaxing, earthy and sensual, patchouli can be overpowering. It is helpful in skin care, particularly rough, chapped or mature skin.

*PEPPERMINT –
mentha piperita – herb.

Cooling, refreshing and invigorating, peppermint is very strong – so only a very little is ever needed. The classic aid to nausea and stomach upsets.

***CAUTION** – use with care.

PETTIGRAIN –
citrus aurantium – tree leaf.

The tonic and astringent properties of pettigrain make this oil useful in skin care preparations and for convalescence.

PINE –
pinus sylvestris – tree.

A stimulating essential oil with effective antiseptic and decongestant properties.

*ROSE –
see main listing for varieties.

Rose has a strong soothing influence on the nervous system and emotions, particularly grief. It has a strong affinity with the female systems and is skin nourishing.

*ROSEMARY –
rosmarinus officinalis – herb.

Rosemary is an effective tonic and stimulant and is generally invigorating, energising and reviving, mentally and physically.

ROSEWOOD –
aniva rosaeaodora – tree.

Rosewood is a very subtle oil, gently uplifting and balancing.

*SANDALWOOD –
santalum album – tree.

Sandalwood is best known for its fortifying and restorative properties. It can promote a warm, relaxed feeling of well being in most situations. It is a good fixative in a blend and is also useful in skin care preparations.

*TEA TREE –
melaleuca alternifolia – tree.

This is known as the "medicine kit in a bottle" due to its highly antiseptic, antifungal, antibacterial uses amongst others. Powerful but safe.

VETIVER –
vetiveria zizanoides – root.

Known for its balancing, grounding and centering properties. Can be revitalising and restorative – a comforting tonic.

VIOLET –
viola odorata – plant.

Reputedly an aphrodisiac with antiseptic and sedative applications.

YARROW –
achillea millefolium – flower.

A cleansing, fortifying and tonic oil, useful in skin and hair care. Can aid digestion and circulation and help regulate female disorders.

*YLANG YLANG –
cananga odorata – flowers.

Ylang Ylang regulates the nervous system and is a known aphrodisiac. It is a very "heady" oil, with warming, sensual and exotic overtones.

CHAPTER NINE

Useful Addresses

Some of the organisations listed are voluntary so please try to enclose a large self-addressed stamped envelope where possible with your enquiry. Some also have local groups or contacts, so check your telephone directory.

Professional Organisations

Aromatherapy Organisations Council (A.O.C.)
3 Latymer Close
Braybrooke
Market Harborough
Leics LE16 8LN
Tel/Fax 01858 434242
(Information, communication and research in Aromatherapy)

The American Aromatherapy Association
PO Box 122
Fair Oaks
CA 95628
U.S.A.

The Aromatherapy Trade Council
PO Box 38
Romford
Essex RM1 2DN

National Association for Holistic
Aromatherapy
219 Carl Street
San Francisco
CA 94117
U.S.A.

International Federation of Aromatherapists
(I.F.A.)
Stamford House
2/4 Chiswick High Road
London W4 1TH
0181 742 2601

International Society of Professional
Aromatherapists (I.S.P.A.)
Hinckley & District Hospital and Health
Centre
The Annex
Mount Road
Hinckley
Leics LE10 1AG
01455 637987

Both the I.F.A. and I.S.P.A. are organisations
that will supply details of qualified aromatherapists in your area, together with registered
schools and colleges.

The Tisserand Aromatherapy Institute
65 Church Road
Hove
East Sussex BN3 2BD
01273 206640
(Contact Hove office for full/part time courses,
mostly held in London & home counties)

London School of Aromatherapy
The Swanfleet Centre
93 Fortess Road
London NW5 1AG

The Raworth Centre
College for Sports Therapy and Natural
Medicine
20–26 South Street
Dorking
Surrey RH4 2HQ
01306 742150
(For full/part time courses both in the U.K.
and overseas)

Aroma Vera Inc
1830 S Robertson Blvd #203
Los Angeles
CA 90035
U.S.A.

European College of Natural Therapies
16 North Parade
Belfast
N. Ireland BT7 2GG
01232 641454

The Israeli College of Natural Health Sciences
c/o PO Box 29627
Tel Aviv 61296
Israel
03 6888838

Australian School of Awareness
PO Box 187
Montrose
3765 Victoria
Australia
010 6137232531

Edinburgh School of Holistic Aromatherapy
6 Roraundle
Monymusk
Aberdeenshire
Scotland AB51 7JL
01467 651238

Sequoia School of Natural Therapies
Unit 2 Williams Court
Trade Street
Penarth Road
Cardiff
South Glamorgan
Wales CF1 5DQ
01222 238599

Kendal College
Milnthorpe Road
Kendal
Cumbria LA9 5AY
01539 724313

Northern School of Aromatherapy
Eastthorpe House
Mirfield
West Yorkshire WF14 8AE
01924 498507

Products

Aromatherapy Products Limited
Newtown Road
Hove
Sussex BN3 7BA
01273 325666

Market leader in supplies of high-quality
essential oils and products, (including organic),
worldwide – for public and professional use.
Fully supportive training packages available for
professional, beautician and retail trade.

Hanny's Health Foods
Corn Exchange Buildings
41a Bondgate Within
Alnwick
Northumberland NE66 4LW
Tel/Fax 01665 604401

Mail order available for Tisserand Essential Oils
and Products and Aveda Esthetique.

Neal's Yard Remedies
15 Neals Yard
Covent Garden
London WC2H 9DP

Remo
Oxford Street
(At Crown Street)
Sydney 2010
Australia

K F Building
3 – Chome 6
Kita Aoyama
Munatu
Tokyo 10
U.S.A.

Aroma Vera Inc.
PO Box 3609
Culver City
CA 90231
U.S.A.
213 973 4253

All the oils distributed by Aroma Vera are extracted from either wild or organically grown plants. The massage oils are specially blended for specific purposes as are the blends for use in diffusers. They also sell diffusers and books.

Ledet Aromatic Oils
PO Box 2354
Fair Oaks
CA 95628
U.S.A.
916 965 7546

Sells a wide range of essential and massage oils, including astrological blends and special blends for use in diffusers. Ledet can provide information on aromatherapy as well as diffusers and books on the subject.

Original Swiss Aromatics
PO Box 606
San Rafael
CA 94915
U.S.A.
415 459 3998
Offers a wide selection of essential oils which are packaged in airtight dropper bottles. It also sells floral waters, face, body, and massage oils, aromatic diffusers, and books on aromatherapy.

Publications

The International Journal of Aromatherapy
PO Box 746
Hove
East Sussex BN3 3XA
01273 772479

Aromatherapy Quarterly (UK)
5 Ranelagh Avenue
London SW19 0BY

Aromatherapy Quarterly (USA)
PO Box 421
Inverness
CA 94937-0421
U.S.A.

Aromatherapy Times
Stamford House
2/4 Chiswick High Road
London W4 1TH

Aromatherapy World
Hinckley & District Hospital and Health
Centre
The Annex
Mount Road
Hinckley
Leics LE10 1AG
01455 637987

***Aromatherapy must be the nicest way to
feel in total harmony – physically, mentally
and emotionally. It is natural, uncomplicated
and works beautifully ... enjoy!

Index

Page references in **bold** indicate an entry in the list of symptoms which refers the user to appropriate oils by name only. Different aspects and degrees of symptoms are indexed by the words used in the text only (e.g. exhaustion/lethargy/tiredness or bereavement/grief/sadness).

E
eczema, 24, 27, 36, 44, 45, **50**
emotions, 43, 46, **50**
energy, **50**
enthusiasm, lack of, 33
essential oils, 3
Eucalyptus (*Eucalyptus globulus*), 30, 62
euphoric oils, **50** *and see* Clary Sage
exhaustion, 42, 43, **50** *and see* fatigue, lethargy, tiredness
expectorant oils, **51** *and see* Benzoin, Eucalyptus, Eucalyptus, Sandalwood, Tea Tree

F
faith, lack of, 31
fatigue, 25, 38, **51**
  mental, 42, **53**
  and see exhaustion, lethargy, tiredness
fear, 31, 36, 43, 59
feet, 17, 29, 39, 44, **51** *and see* athlete's foot
femininity, **51**
Fennel (*Foeniculum vulgare*), 62
fevers, 27, 62 *and see* colds, influenza
fleas, **51**
fluid retention, 32, **51** *and see* oedema
focus of thoughts, 26, **51**, 59, 61 *and see* clarity
fortifying oils *see* Cedarwood, Frankincense, Rosemary, Sandalwood, Yarrow
Frankincense (*Boswellia thurifera*), 31, 62–3
frigidity, 33, **51**
frustration, 38, 46, **51**
fungi *see* athlete's foot

G
gargles 13, **51** *and see* throats
gastritis, 32
Gattefossé, René, 1
Geranium (*Pelargonium graveolens/odoratissimum*), 32, 63
german measles **51** *and see* measles
glands, adrenal, 43
Ginger (*Zingiber officinale*), 63
gout, 23, 27, **51**
Grapefruit (*Citrus paradisi*), 63
grapeseed oil, 10
grief, 31, 38, 41, **51**, 67
guilt, **52**
gum infections, 44

H
haemorrhoids, 29, 44, **52**
hair treatments, 15–16, 44, 68
  and see dandruff
hangovers, 35, 40, 42, **52**
harmonising oils *see* Geranium, Lavender
head lice *see* lice
headaches, 30, 35, 36, 38, 40, **52**
heat bumps/rash, 36, 44, **52** *and see* rashes
herpes, 24, 44, **52** *and see* cold sores
hibernation, 42
holistic aromatherapy, xii–xiii
hopelessness, 31, 38, 41, **52**
hormones, 32, **52**
humility, 43
hyperactivity, 32, 36
hypertension, 38, **52** *and see* blood pressure
hypoactivity, 32
Hyssop (*Hyssopus officinalis*), 63
hysteria, 36

I
immune system, 36, 43, **52**, 65
impatience, 36
impotence, 33
indecision, 42
indifference, 25
indigestion, 38, 39, **52** *and see* digestive problems
inertness, 42
infections, 23, 44, **52**
inflammation, 27, 44, **50**, **52** *and see* oedema
influenza, 23, 30, 43, 44, 45, **52** *and see* colds, fevers
inhalations, 12–13
insect bites/stings, 36, 44, **52** *and see* bites, stings
insect repellent, 30, 44, **53**, 61
insecurity, 31
insomnia, 36, 38, **53**, 64 *and see* sleep
introversion, 46
invigorating oils *see* Peppermint *and see* stimulating oils
irritability, 31, 36, 38, **53**

J
Jasmine (*Jasminum officinale/grandiflorum*), 3, 33–4, 63
jealousy, 36, 46, **53**
jojoba oil, 10
Juniper (*juniperus communis*), 35, 64